THIS PLANNER

Belongs To:

Dedication:

This book is dedicated to all the amazing
New Moms in the world.

You are my inspiration in producing books and I'm excited
to be able to help in the planning of all parts of your
pregnancy!

How to Use this book

The purpose of this book is to keep all your pregnancy plans and ideas organized in one easy to find spot. Here are some simple guidelines to follow so you can make the most of using this book:

1. Use the fill in the blank prompt pages in this planner to help navigate your pregnancy from bump to delivery. This will make it easy for you to keep everything organized!

2. The first Pregnancy Planner section is for you to write the "Birth Plan" of your little one's arrival.

3. Most ideas are inspired by something we have seen. Use the "Doctor and Prenatal Appointment Tracker" section to write down all your appointments and the results of that appointment.

4. The "Baby Shower Memories" section is for you to detail out a description of your fun Baby Shower day.
Don't worry, there will be more space for you to go in-depth with space for notes.

5. Some keepsake memories that you love to remember, are the "Fetal Movement Tracker" is great for that. more memories you will record and make notes about!

6. Flip the page over and this is where your "Baby Shopping List" begins.

7. Write down the action steps you need to complete your pregnancy plans, and "First, Second, Third Trimester" thoughts and feelings.

8. The "Baby Bump Photo Layouts" section is so you can visually track your pregnancy and be inspired later after the baby is born that you finished!

9. Use The "Nursery Planner" to find the perfect baby room layout, and make it a beautiful room for baby's arrival.

And finally pages with BLANK lines for you to journal about your new life with baby, brainstorm and watch your plans unfold...

Have fun!

I'm PREGNANT!

DUE DATE

How I found out

My reaction

WHAT I AM MOST EXCITED ABOUT

WHO I TOLD FIRST

WHAT I WANT YOU TO KNOW

MY BIRTH PLAN Ideas

WHO I WANT IN THE DELIVERY ROOM:

mom
michael

TYPE OF BIRTH

☑ VAGINAL   ☑ WATER BIRTH

☐ C-SECTION   ☐ VBAC

THOUGHTS ABOUT BIRTH AND WHAT IS MOST IMPORTANT TO ME

GETTING READY FOR THE BIG DAY: TO DO

NOTES & IDEAS (lighting, music, etc.)

Keep track of how you're feeling every week of your pregnancy.

1	2	3	4	5	6	7
8	9	10	11	12	13	14
15	16	17	18	19	20	21
22 first kick	23	24	25	26	27	28
29	30	31	32	33	34	35
36	37	38	39	40		

APPOINTMENT Tracker

Keep track of your pre-natal classes and doctor appointments.

DATE	TIME	ADDRESS	PURPOSE

BABY SHOPPING List

Start planning for the arrival of your baby by using the shopping list below.

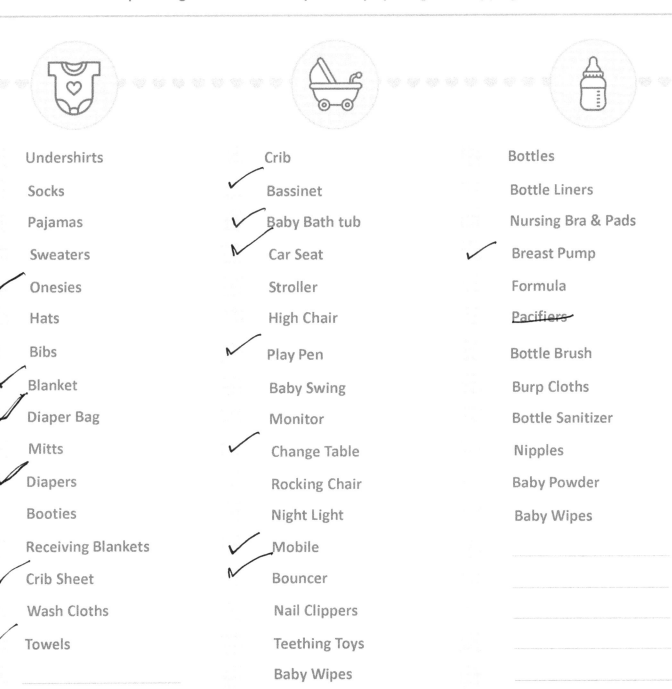

Undershirts	Crib	Bottles
Socks	✓ Bassinet	Bottle Liners
Pajamas	✓ Baby Bath tub	Nursing Bra & Pads
Sweaters	✓ Car Seat	✓ Breast Pump
✓ Onesies	Stroller	Formula
Hats	High Chair	~~Pacifiers~~
Bibs	✓ Play Pen	Bottle Brush
✓ Blanket	Baby Swing	Burp Cloths
✓ Diaper Bag	Monitor	Bottle Sanitizer
Mitts	✓ Change Table	Nipples
✓ Diapers	Rocking Chair	Baby Powder
Booties	Night Light	Baby Wipes
Receiving Blankets	✓ Mobile	
✓ Crib Sheet	✓ Bouncer	
Wash Cloths	Nail Clippers	
✓ Towels	Teething Toys	
	Baby Wipes	
	Diaper Pail	

Weight PREGNANCY Tracker

Weight Tracker Chart

It's important to keep track of your weight throughout your pregnancy.
Record your weight in the chart below every week, starting at week 4.

WEEKLY WEIGHT TRACKER

4	12	20	28	36
5	13	21	29	37
6	14	22	30	38
7	15	23	31	39
8	16	24	32	40
9	17	25	33	
10	18	26	34	
11	19	27	35	

NOTE According to the American Pregnancy Association, pregnant women should consume up to 300 more calories a day. Further, healthy eating is critical to your baby's development which means you should make sure to maintain a well-balanced diet, high in nutrients and proteins.

HEALTHY FOOD Ideas

VEGETABLES & LOW SUGAR FRUIT	PROTEINS	COMPLEX CARBS	HEALTHY FATS	SUPPLEMENTS
Leafy greens (spinach, etc.)	Organic meat	Beets	Avocado	Vitamin D
Broccoli	Liver	Carrots	Olive Oil	Fish Oil
Cauliflower	Bone Broth	Sweet Potatoes	Coconut Oil	Algae Oil
Cabbage	Beans	Yams	Yogurt	Probiotics
Asparagus	Lentils	Parsnips	Almonds	Ginger Pills
Cucumber	Flax Seed	Turnips	Mixed Nuts	Licorice Root
Mushrooms	Pumpkin Seed	Pumpkin	Soybean	Magnesium
Celery	Chia Seed	Buckwheat	Olives	Krill Oil
Radish	Salmon	Brown Rice	Nut butter	Iron Pills
Grapefruit & Melon	Herring	Squash		
Berries (all kinds)				
Peaches (with skin)				

PRE-NATAL Visits

Important Dates

Keep track of your pre-natal appointments and include a summary of each visit.

	Summary of Appointment
Date	
How far along?	
Your Weight	
Blood Pressure	
Fetal Heart Rate	
Doctor	
NOTES:	

Next Appointment.:

	Summary of Appointment
Date	
How far along?	
Your Weight	
Blood Pressure	
Fetal Heart Rate	
Doctor	
NOTES:	

Next Appointment.:

	Summary of Appointment
Date	
How far along?	
Your Weight	
Blood Pressure	
Fetal Heart Rate	
Doctor	
NOTES:	

Next Appointment.:

1-13 Weeks

FIRST Trimester

HOW I FELT DURING MY FIRST TRIMESTER

MY FAVORITE MEMORIES

SYMPTOMS & CRAVINGS

ENERGY

SLEEP

CRAVINGS

MOODS

TO DO LIST: 1st TRIMESTER

FIRST TRIMESTER Photos

MEMORIES ARE FOREVER

14-27 Weeks

SECOND Trimester

♥♥♥ ♥♥♥ ♥♥♥ ♥♥♥ ♥♥♥ ♥♥♥ ♥♥♥ ♥♥♥

HOW I FELT DURING MY SECOND TRIMESTER

....
....
....
....

MY FAVORITE MEMORIES

....
....
....
....

SYMPTOMS & CRAVINGS

....
....
....
....
....
....
....
....

ENERGY
♥ ♥ ♥ ♥ ♥ ♥

SLEEP
♥ ♥ ♥ ♥ ♥ ♥

CRAVINGS
♥ ♥ ♥ ♥ ♥ ♥

MOODS
♥ ♥ ♥ ♥ ♥ ♥

TO DO LIST: 2nd TRIMESTER

_____
_____
_____
_____
_____
_____
_____
_____
_____
_____
_____
_____

SECOND TRIMESTER Photos

MEMORIES ARE FOREVER

28-40 Weeks

THIRD Trimester

HOW I FELT DURING MY THIRD TRIMESTER

MY FAVORITE MEMORIES

SYMPTOMS & CRAVINGS

ENERGY

SLEEP

CRAVINGS

MOODS

TO DO LIST: 3rd TRIMESTER

THIRD TRIMESTER Photos

MEMORIES ARE FOREVER

MY BABY Shower

BABY SHOWER PHOTOS

GAMES PLAYED

ON THE MENU

HIGHLIGHTS & MEMORIES

MY BABY Shower Gifts

Keep track of your baby shower gifts and send thank you notes

NAME	GIFT	ADDRESS	SENT?

NURSERY Planner

COLOR SCHEME IDEAS:

ITEM TO PURCHASE	PRICE	NOTES

FURNITURE IDEAS

DECORATIVE IDEAS

BABY NAME Ideas

TOP 3 BOY NAMES

NAME
MEANINGS

TOP 3 GIRL NAMES

NAME
MEANINGS

BABY NAME RESOURCES (LIST YOUR FAVORITE PARENTING & PREGNANCY WEBSITES):		

OTHER BOY NAME POSSIBILITIES	OTHER GIRL NAME POSSIBILITES

HOSPITAL Checklist

FOR ME	FOR PARTNER	FOR BABY

PREGNANCY SHOPPING List

BABY CLOTHING

SUPPLIES/MEDICATION

FURNITURE/TOYS

FIRST TRIMESTER SHOPPING

SECOND TRIMESTER SHOPPING

THIRD TRIMESTER SHOPPING

Tracker FETAL Movement

Starting around week 16, keep track of when you feel your baby move.

WEEK 16	TIME	NOTES
MON		
TUE		
WED		
THU		
FRI		
SAT		
SUN		

WEEK 17	TIME	NOTES
MON		
TUE		
WED		
THU		
FRI		
SAT		
SUN		

WEEK 18	TIME	NOTES
MON		
TUE		
WED		
THU		
FRI		
SAT		
SUN		

WEEK 19	TIME	NOTES
MON		
TUE		
WED		
THU		
FRI		
SAT		
SUN		

WEEK 20	TIME	NOTES
MON		
TUE		
WED		
THU		
FRI		
SAT		
SUN		

WEEK 21	TIME	NOTES
MON		
TUE		
WED		
THU		
FRI		
SAT		
SUN		

First kick

WEEK 22	TIME	NOTES
MON		
TUE		
WED		
THU		
FRI		
SAT		
SUN		

WEEK 23	TIME	NOTES
MON		
TUE		
WED		
THU		
FRI		
SAT		
SUN		

WEEK 24	TIME	NOTES
MON		
TUE		
WED		
THU		
FRI		
SAT		
SUN		

Tracker

FETAL Movement

WEEK 25	TIME	NOTES
MON		
TUE		
WED		
THU		
FRI		
SAT		
SUN		

WEEK 26	TIME	NOTES
MON		
TUE		
WED		
THU		
FRI		
SAT		
SUN		

WEEK 27	TIME	NOTES
MON		
TUE		
WED		
THU		
FRI		
SAT		
SUN		

WEEK 28	TIME	NOTES
MON		
TUE		
WED		
THU		
FRI		
SAT		
SUN		

WEEK 29	TIME	NOTES
MON		
TUE		
WED		
THU		
FRI		
SAT		
SUN		

WEEK 30	TIME	NOTES
MON		
TUE		
WED		
THU		
FRI		
SAT		
SUN		

WEEK 31	TIME	NOTES
MON		
TUE		
WED		
THU		
FRI		
SAT		
SUN		

WEEK 32	TIME	NOTES
MON		
TUE		
WED		
THU		
FRI		
SAT		
SUN		

WEEK 33	TIME	NOTES
MON		
TUE		
WED		
THU		
FRI		
SAT		
SUN		

Tracker FETAL Movement

WEEK 34	TIME	NOTES
MON		
TUE		
WED		
THU		
FRI		
SAT		
SUN		

WEEK 35	TIME	NOTES
MON		
TUE		
WED		
THU		
FRI		
SAT		
SUN		

WEEK 36	TIME	NOTES
MON		
TUE		
WED		
THU		
FRI		
SAT		
SUN		

WEEK 37	TIME	NOTES
MON		
TUE		
WED		
THU		
FRI		
SAT		
SUN		

WEEK 38	TIME	NOTES
MON		
TUE		
WED		
THU		
FRI		
SAT		
SUN		

WEEK 39	TIME	NOTES
MON		
TUE		
WED		
THU		
FRI		
SAT		
SUN		

WEEK 40	TIME	NOTES
MON		
TUE		
WED		
THU		
FRI		
SAT		
SUN		

NOTES		

Week 4

PREGNANCY Journal

Your baby is the size of a poppy seed!

TOTAL WEIGHT GAIN

BELLY MEASUREMENT

BABY BUMP PHOTO

WEEKLY REFLECTIONS

SYMPTOMS & CRAVINGS

WHAT I WANT TO REMEMBER MOST

Dear Baby

I'M MOST EXCITED ABOUT

I'M MOST NERVOUS ABOUT

Dear Baby

PREGNANCY Journal

TODAY'S DATE

WEEKS PREGNANT

HOW I'M FEELING TODAY

What I want you to know

Week 5 PREGNANCY Journal

Your baby is the size of a peppercorn!

TOTAL WEIGHT GAIN

BELLY MEASUREMENT

WEEKLY REFLECTIONS

SYMPTOMS & CRAVINGS

WHAT I WANT TO REMEMBER MOST

I'M MOST EXCITED ABOUT

I'M MOST NERVOUS ABOUT

BABY BUMP PHOTO

Dear Baby

Dear Baby

PREGNANCY Journal

TODAY'S DATE

WEEKS PREGNANT

HOW I'M FEELING TODAY

What I want you to know

Week 6

PREGNANCY Journal

Your baby is the size of a sweet pea!

TOTAL WEIGHT GAIN

BELLY MEASUREMENT

BABY BUMP PHOTO

WEEKLY REFLECTIONS

SYMPTOMS & CRAVINGS

WHAT I WANT TO REMEMBER MOST

I'M MOST EXCITED ABOUT

I'M MOST NERVOUS ABOUT

Dear Baby

Dear Baby

PREGNANCY Journal

TODAY'S DATE

WEEKS PREGNANT

HOW I'M FEELING TODAY

What I want you to know

Week 7

PREGNANCY Journal

Your baby is the size of a blueberry!

TOTAL WEIGHT GAIN

BELLY MEASUREMENT

BABY BUMP PHOTO

WEEKLY REFLECTIONS

SYMPTOMS & CRAVINGS

WHAT I WANT TO REMEMBER MOST

Dear Baby

I'M MOST EXCITED ABOUT

I'M MOST NERVOUS ABOUT

Dear Baby

PREGNANCY Journal

TODAY'S DATE

WEEKS PREGNANT

HOW I'M FEELING TODAY

What I want you to know

Week 8

PREGNANCY Journal

Your baby is the size of a raspberry!

TOTAL WEIGHT GAIN

BELLY MEASUREMENT

BABY BUMP PHOTO

WEEKLY REFLECTIONS

SYMPTOMS & CRAVINGS

WHAT I WANT TO REMEMBER MOST

I'M MOST EXCITED ABOUT

I'M MOST NERVOUS ABOUT

Dear Baby

Dear Baby

PREGNANCY Journal

TODAY'S DATE

WEEKS PREGNANT

HOW I'M FEELING TODAY

What I want you to know

Week 9

PREGNANCY Journal

Your baby is the size of a grape!

TOTAL WEIGHT GAIN

BELLY MEASUREMENT

BABY BUMP PHOTO

WEEKLY REFLECTIONS

SYMPTOMS & CRAVINGS

WHAT I WANT TO REMEMBER MOST

I'M MOST EXCITED ABOUT

I'M MOST NERVOUS ABOUT

Dear Baby

Dear Baby

PREGNANCY Journal

TODAY'S DATE

WEEKS PREGNANT

HOW I'M FEELING TODAY

What I want you to know

Week 10

PREGNANCY Journal

Your baby is the size of a prune!

TOTAL WEIGHT GAIN

BELLY MEASUREMENT

BABY BUMP PHOTO

WEEKLY REFLECTIONS

SYMPTOMS & CRAVINGS

WHAT I WANT TO REMEMBER MOST

I'M MOST EXCITED ABOUT

I'M MOST NERVOUS ABOUT

Dear Baby

Dear Baby

PREGNANCY Journal

TODAY'S DATE

WEEKS PREGNANT

HOW I'M FEELING TODAY

What I want you to know

Week 11

PREGNANCY Journal

Your baby is the size of a lime!

TOTAL WEIGHT GAIN

BELLY MEASUREMENT

BABY BUMP PHOTO

WEEKLY REFLECTIONS

SYMPTOMS & CRAVINGS

WHAT I WANT TO REMEMBER MOST

Dear Baby

I'M MOST EXCITED ABOUT

I'M MOST NERVOUS ABOUT

Dear Baby

PREGNANCY Journal

TODAY'S DATE

WEEKS PREGNANT

HOW I'M FEELING TODAY

What I want you to know

PREGNANCY Journal

Your baby is the size of a plum!

TOTAL WEIGHT GAIN

BELLY MEASUREMENT

BABY BUMP PHOTO

WEEKLY REFLECTIONS

SYMPTOMS & CRAVINGS

WHAT I WANT TO REMEMBER MOST

Dear Baby

I'M MOST EXCITED ABOUT

I'M MOST NERVOUS ABOUT

ULTRASOUND PHOTO

ULTRASOUND RESULTS

BABY'S LENGTH:

BABY'S WEIGHT:

BPD:

DUE DATE:

Notes

Dear Baby

PREGNANCY Journal

TODAY'S DATE

WEEKS PREGNANT

HOW I'M FEELING TODAY

What I want you to know

Week 13 — PREGNANCY Journal

Your baby is the size of a peach!

TOTAL WEIGHT GAIN

BELLY MEASUREMENT

BABY BUMP PHOTO

WEEKLY REFLECTIONS

SYMPTOMS & CRAVINGS

WHAT I WANT TO REMEMBER MOST

I'M MOST EXCITED ABOUT

I'M MOST NERVOUS ABOUT

Dear Baby

Dear Baby

PREGNANCY Journal

TODAY'S DATE

WEEKS PREGNANT

HOW I'M FEELING TODAY

What I want you to know

PREGNANCY Journal

Your baby is the size of a lemon!

TOTAL WEIGHT GAIN

BELLY MEASUREMENT

BABY BUMP PHOTO

WEEKLY REFLECTIONS

SYMPTOMS & CRAVINGS

WHAT I WANT TO REMEMBER MOST

I'M MOST EXCITED ABOUT

I'M MOST NERVOUS ABOUT

Dear Baby

Dear Baby

PREGNANCY Journal

TODAY'S DATE

WEEKS PREGNANT

HOW I'M FEELING TODAY

What I want you to know

PREGNANCY Journal

Your baby is the size of an apple!

TOTAL WEIGHT GAIN

BELLY MEASUREMENT

BABY BUMP PHOTO

WEEKLY REFLECTIONS

SYMPTOMS & CRAVINGS

WHAT I WANT TO REMEMBER MOST

I'M MOST EXCITED ABOUT

I'M MOST NERVOUS ABOUT

Dear Baby

Dear Baby

PREGNANCY Journal

TODAY'S DATE

WEEKS PREGNANT

HOW I'M FEELING TODAY

What I want you to know

Week 16 | PREGNANCY Journal

Your baby is the size of an avocado!

TOTAL WEIGHT GAIN

BELLY MEASUREMENT

BABY BUMP PHOTO

WEEKLY REFLECTIONS

SYMPTOMS & CRAVINGS

WHAT I WANT TO REMEMBER MOST

I'M MOST EXCITED ABOUT

I'M MOST NERVOUS ABOUT

Dear Baby

Dear Baby

PREGNANCY Journal

TODAY'S DATE

WEEKS PREGNANT

HOW I'M FEELING TODAY

What I want you to know

Week 17

PREGNANCY Journal

Your baby is the size of a pear!

TOTAL WEIGHT GAIN

BELLY MEASUREMENT

BABY BUMP PHOTO

WEEKLY REFLECTIONS

SYMPTOMS & CRAVINGS

WHAT I WANT TO REMEMBER MOST

I'M MOST EXCITED ABOUT

I'M MOST NERVOUS ABOUT

Dear Baby

Dear Baby

PREGNANCY Journal

TODAY'S DATE

WEEKS PREGNANT

HOW I'M FEELING TODAY

What I want you to know

Week 18

PREGNANCY Journal

Your baby is the size of a sweet potato!

TOTAL WEIGHT GAIN

BELLY MEASUREMENT

BABY BUMP PHOTO

WEEKLY REFLECTIONS

SYMPTOMS & CRAVINGS

WHAT I WANT TO REMEMBER MOST

I'M MOST EXCITED ABOUT

I'M MOST NERVOUS ABOUT

Dear Baby

Dear Baby

PREGNANCY Journal

TODAY'S DATE

WEEKS PREGNANT

HOW I'M FEELING TODAY

What I want you to know

Week 19

PREGNANCY Journal

Your baby is the size of a mango!

TOTAL WEIGHT GAIN

BELLY MEASUREMENT

BABY BUMP PHOTO

WEEKLY REFLECTIONS

SYMPTOMS & CRAVINGS

WHAT I WANT TO REMEMBER MOST

Dear Baby

I'M MOST EXCITED ABOUT

I'M MOST NERVOUS ABOUT

Dear Baby

PREGNANCY Journal

TODAY'S DATE

WEEKS PREGNANT

HOW I'M FEELING TODAY

What I want you to know

PREGNANCY Journal

Your baby is the size of a banana!

TOTAL WEIGHT GAIN

BELLY MEASUREMENT

BABY BUMP PHOTO

WEEKLY REFLECTIONS

SYMPTOMS & CRAVINGS

WHAT I WANT TO REMEMBER MOST

I'M MOST EXCITED ABOUT

I'M MOST NERVOUS ABOUT

Dear Baby

20 WEEKS

ULTRASOUND Scan

ULTRASOUND PHOTO

ULTRASOUND RESULTS

BABY'S LENGTH:

BABY'S WEIGHT:

BPD:

DUE DATE:

Notes

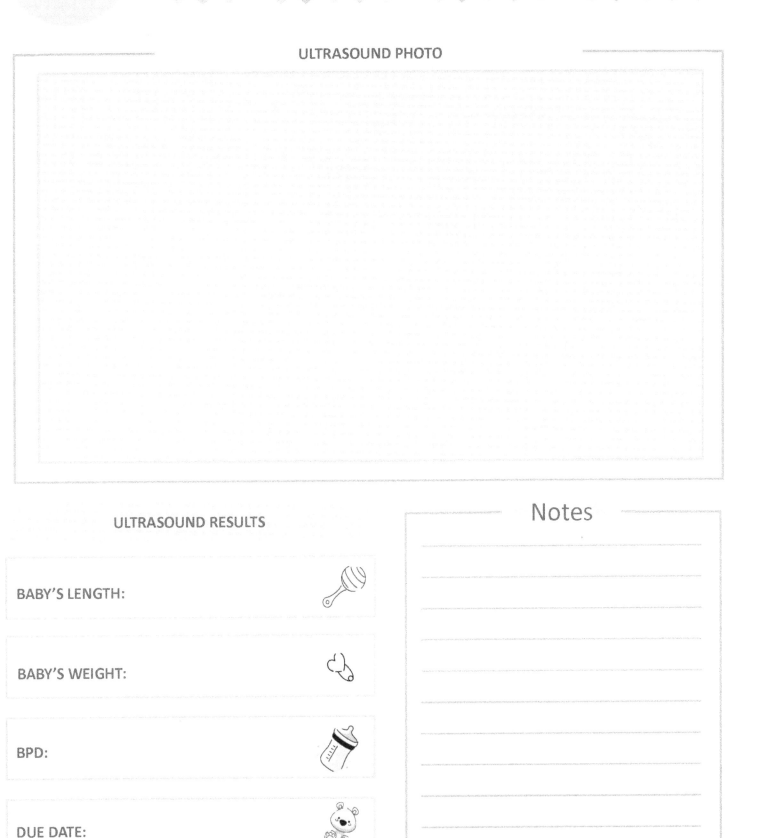

Dear Baby

PREGNANCY Journal

TODAY'S DATE

WEEKS PREGNANT

HOW I'M FEELING TODAY

What I want you to know

PREGNANCY Journal

Your baby is the size of a carrot!

TOTAL WEIGHT GAIN

BELLY MEASUREMENT

BABY BUMP PHOTO

WEEKLY REFLECTIONS

SYMPTOMS & CRAVINGS

WHAT I WANT TO REMEMBER MOST

I'M MOST EXCITED ABOUT

I'M MOST NERVOUS ABOUT

Dear Baby

Dear Baby

PREGNANCY Journal

TODAY'S DATE

WEEKS PREGNANT

HOW I'M FEELING TODAY

What I want you to know

PREGNANCY Journal

Your baby is the size of a papaya!

TOTAL WEIGHT GAIN

BELLY MEASUREMENT

BABY BUMP PHOTO

WEEKLY REFLECTIONS

SYMPTOMS & CRAVINGS

WHAT I WANT TO REMEMBER MOST

Dear Baby

I'M MOST EXCITED ABOUT

I'M MOST NERVOUS ABOUT

Dear Baby

PREGNANCY Journal

TODAY'S DATE

WEEKS PREGNANT

HOW I'M FEELING TODAY

What I want you to know

PREGNANCY Journal

Your baby is the size of a grapefruit!

TOTAL WEIGHT GAIN

BELLY MEASUREMENT

BABY BUMP PHOTO

WEEKLY REFLECTIONS

SYMPTOMS & CRAVINGS

WHAT I WANT TO REMEMBER MOST

I'M MOST EXCITED ABOUT

I'M MOST NERVOUS ABOUT

Dear Baby

Dear Baby

PREGNANCY Journal

TODAY'S DATE

WEEKS PREGNANT

HOW I'M FEELING TODAY

What I want you to know

Week 24

PREGNANCY Journal

Your baby is the size of a cantaloupe!

TOTAL WEIGHT GAIN

BELLY MEASUREMENT

WEEKLY REFLECTIONS

SYMPTOMS & CRAVINGS

WHAT I WANT TO REMEMBER MOST

I'M MOST EXCITED ABOUT

I'M MOST NERVOUS ABOUT

BABY BUMP PHOTO

Dear Baby

Dear Baby

PREGNANCY Journal

TODAY'S DATE

WEEKS PREGNANT

HOW I'M FEELING TODAY

What I want you to know

Week 25

PREGNANCY Journal

TOTAL WEIGHT GAIN

BELLY MEASUREMENT

Your baby is the size of a cauliflower!

WEEKLY REFLECTIONS

BABY BUMP PHOTO

SYMPTOMS & CRAVINGS

WHAT I WANT TO REMEMBER MOST

I'M MOST EXCITED ABOUT

I'M MOST NERVOUS ABOUT

Dear Baby

Dear Baby

PREGNANCY Journal

TODAY'S DATE

WEEKS PREGNANT

HOW I'M FEELING TODAY

What I want you to know

Week 26

PREGNANCY Journal

Your baby is the size of a head of lettuce!

TOTAL WEIGHT GAIN

BELLY MEASUREMENT

BABY BUMP PHOTO

WEEKLY REFLECTIONS

SYMPTOMS & CRAVINGS

WHAT I WANT TO REMEMBER MOST

I'M MOST EXCITED ABOUT

I'M MOST NERVOUS ABOUT

Dear Baby

Dear Baby

PREGNANCY Journal

TODAY'S DATE

WEEKS PREGNANT

HOW I'M FEELING TODAY

What I want you to know

Week 27

PREGNANCY Journal

Your baby is the size of a rutabaga!

TOTAL WEIGHT GAIN

BELLY MEASUREMENT

BABY BUMP PHOTO

WEEKLY REFLECTIONS

SYMPTOMS & CRAVINGS

Dear Baby

WHAT I WANT TO REMEMBER MOST

I'M MOST EXCITED ABOUT

I'M MOST NERVOUS ABOUT

Dear Baby

PREGNANCY Journal

TODAY'S DATE

WEEKS PREGNANT

HOW I'M FEELING TODAY

What I want you to know

PREGNANCY Journal

Your baby is the size of an eggplant!

**TOTAL
WEIGHT GAIN**

BELLY MEASUREMENT

BABY BUMP PHOTO

WEEKLY REFLECTIONS

SYMPTOMS & CRAVINGS

WHAT I WANT TO REMEMBER MOST

I'M MOST EXCITED ABOUT

I'M MOST NERVOUS ABOUT

Dear Baby

Dear Baby

PREGNANCY Journal

TODAY'S DATE

WEEKS PREGNANT

HOW I'M FEELING TODAY

What I want you to know

Week 29

PREGNANCY Journal

Your baby is the size of acorn squash!

TOTAL WEIGHT GAIN

BELLY MEASUREMENT

BABY BUMP PHOTO

WEEKLY REFLECTIONS

SYMPTOMS & CRAVINGS

WHAT I WANT TO REMEMBER MOST

I'M MOST EXCITED ABOUT

I'M MOST NERVOUS ABOUT

Dear Baby

Dear Baby

PREGNANCY Journal

TODAY'S DATE

WEEKS PREGNANT

HOW I'M FEELING TODAY

What I want you to know

PREGNANCY Journal

TOTAL WEIGHT GAIN

BELLY MEASUREMENT

Your baby is the size of a cucumber!

BABY BUMP PHOTO

WEEKLY REFLECTIONS

SYMPTOMS & CRAVINGS

WHAT I WANT TO REMEMBER MOST

I'M MOST EXCITED ABOUT

I'M MOST NERVOUS ABOUT

Dear Baby

Dear Baby

PREGNANCY Journal

TODAY'S DATE

WEEKS PREGNANT

HOW I'M FEELING TODAY

What I want you to know

Week 31

PREGNANCY Journal

Your baby is the size of a pineapple!

TOTAL WEIGHT GAIN

BELLY MEASUREMENT

BABY BUMP PHOTO

WEEKLY REFLECTIONS

SYMPTOMS & CRAVINGS

WHAT I WANT TO REMEMBER MOST

Dear Baby

I'M MOST EXCITED ABOUT

I'M MOST NERVOUS ABOUT

Dear Baby

PREGNANCY Journal

TODAY'S DATE

WEEKS PREGNANT

HOW I'M FEELING TODAY

What I want you to know

Week 32

PREGNANCY Journal

Your baby is the size of a squash!

TOTAL WEIGHT GAIN

BELLY MEASUREMENT

BABY BUMP PHOTO

WEEKLY REFLECTIONS

SYMPTOMS & CRAVINGS

WHAT I WANT TO REMEMBER MOST

I'M MOST EXCITED ABOUT

I'M MOST NERVOUS ABOUT

Dear Baby

Dear Baby

PREGNANCY Journal

TODAY'S DATE

WEEKS PREGNANT

HOW I'M FEELING TODAY

What I want you to know

PREGNANCY Journal

Your baby is the size of a durian!

TOTAL WEIGHT GAIN

BELLY MEASUREMENT

BABY BUMP PHOTO

WEEKLY REFLECTIONS

SYMPTOMS & CRAVINGS

WHAT I WANT TO REMEMBER MOST

Dear Baby

I'M MOST EXCITED ABOUT

I'M MOST NERVOUS ABOUT

Dear Baby

PREGNANCY Journal

TODAY'S DATE

WEEKS PREGNANT

HOW I'M FEELING TODAY

What I want you to know

Week 34

PREGNANCY Journal

Your baby is the size of a butternut squash!

TOTAL WEIGHT GAIN

BELLY MEASUREMENT

BABY BUMP PHOTO

WEEKLY REFLECTIONS

SYMPTOMS & CRAVINGS

WHAT I WANT TO REMEMBER MOST

I'M MOST EXCITED ABOUT

I'M MOST NERVOUS ABOUT

Dear Baby

Dear Baby

PREGNANCY Journal

TODAY'S DATE

WEEKS PREGNANT

HOW I'M FEELING TODAY

What I want you to know

Week 35

PREGNANCY Journal

Your baby is the size of a coconut!

TOTAL WEIGHT GAIN

BELLY MEASUREMENT

BABY BUMP PHOTO

WEEKLY REFLECTIONS

SYMPTOMS & CRAVINGS

WHAT I WANT TO REMEMBER MOST

Dear Baby

I'M MOST EXCITED ABOUT

I'M MOST NERVOUS ABOUT

Dear Baby

PREGNANCY Journal

TODAY'S DATE

WEEKS PREGNANT

HOW I'M FEELING TODAY

What I want you to know

PREGNANCY Journal

Your baby is the size of a honeydew melon!

TOTAL WEIGHT GAIN

BELLY MEASUREMENT

BABY BUMP PHOTO

WEEKLY REFLECTIONS

SYMPTOMS & CRAVINGS

WHAT I WANT TO REMEMBER MOST

I'M MOST EXCITED ABOUT

I'M MOST NERVOUS ABOUT

Dear Baby

Dear Baby

PREGNANCY Journal

TODAY'S DATE

WEEKS PREGNANT

HOW I'M FEELING TODAY

What I want you to know

Your baby is the size of a Winter Melon!

TOTAL WEIGHT GAIN

BELLY MEASUREMENT

BABY BUMP PHOTO

WEEKLY REFLECTIONS

SYMPTOMS & CRAVINGS

WHAT I WANT TO REMEMBER MOST

Dear Baby

I'M MOST EXCITED ABOUT

I'M MOST NERVOUS ABOUT

Dear Baby

PREGNANCY Journal

TODAY'S DATE

WEEKS PREGNANT

HOW I'M FEELING TODAY

What I want you to know

PREGNANCY Journal

Your baby is the size of a pumpkin!

TOTAL WEIGHT GAIN

BELLY MEASUREMENT

BABY BUMP PHOTO

WEEKLY REFLECTIONS

SYMPTOMS & CRAVINGS

WHAT I WANT TO REMEMBER MOST

I'M MOST EXCITED ABOUT

I'M MOST NERVOUS ABOUT

Dear Baby

Dear Baby

PREGNANCY Journal

TODAY'S DATE

WEEKS PREGNANT

HOW I'M FEELING TODAY

What I want you to know

Week 39

PREGNANCY Journal

Your baby is the size of a watermelon!

TOTAL WEIGHT GAIN

BELLY MEASUREMENT

BABY BUMP PHOTO

WEEKLY REFLECTIONS

SYMPTOMS & CRAVINGS

WHAT I WANT TO REMEMBER MOST

I'M MOST EXCITED ABOUT

I'M MOST NERVOUS ABOUT

Dear Baby

Dear Baby

PREGNANCY Journal

TODAY'S DATE

WEEKS PREGNANT

HOW I'M FEELING TODAY

What I want you to know

PREGNANCY Journal

Your baby is the size of a jack fruit!

TOTAL WEIGHT GAIN

BELLY MEASUREMENT

BABY BUMP PHOTO

WEEKLY REFLECTIONS

SYMPTOMS & CRAVINGS

WHAT I WANT TO REMEMBER MOST

I'M MOST EXCITED ABOUT

I'M MOST NERVOUS ABOUT

Dear Baby

Dear Baby

PREGNANCY Journal

TODAY'S DATE

WEEKS PREGNANT

HOW I'M FEELING TODAY

What I want you to know

Printed in the USA
CPSIA information can be obtained
at www.ICGtesting.com
LVHW080803241024
794662LV00018B/203